GETTING

MW00903840

Dr. Howard Peiper

Copyright© 2005 by Howard Peiper All Rights Reserved

No part of this book may be reproduced in any form without the written consent of the publisher.

Categories: 1. Health 2. Nitric Oxide Printed in the U.S.A.

Revised 2017

Getting to Know NO is not intended as medical advice. It is written solely for informational and educational purposes. Please consult a health professional should the need for one be indicated. Because there is always some risk involved, the author and publisher are not responsible for any adverse effects or consequences resulting from the use of any of the suggestions, preparations or methods described in this book. The publisher does not advocate the use of any particular diet or health program, but believes the information presented in this book should be available to the public.

Published by

Walk the Talk Productions

(760) 902 3343

CONTENTS

AUTHOR'S STATEMENT

I believe that in the next one to three years most people will be using a nitric oxide supplement for cardiovascular health, as well as to enhance metabolism, renew strength and endurance, and experience overall improvement in health. In fact, nitric oxide may stop, and even reverse, the build-up of arterial plaque. The future is now, so take charge of your health.

Howard Peiper, N.D.

July 2017

"Nitric Oxide could change scientists' view of how proteins work together to drive the cellular machinery"
Jonathan S. Stamler, M.D
Duke University

CHAPTER 1

NITRIC OXIDE

The Biggest Little Molecule in Biology!

We live in an age of exhilarating medical discoveries. Scientific breakthroughs occur routinely and " miracle drugs" rise and fall in popularity. However, this booklet is not about the latest magic bullet that will cure everything that ails you. It is about a natural substance, nitric oxide (NO) that has emerged in past decades as one of medicine's greatest untold success stories and one of the human body's best allies in its intrinsic quest for wellness.

Nitric oxide (NO), is a free radical gas that is a powerful regulator of circulation (it is an endogenous vasodilator) and a neurotransmitter (it helps in the processing of nerve signals as they cross synapses. L-arginine, one of the 20 amino acids that make up protein, is the only amino acid that generates significant amounts of nitric oxide. Nitric oxide initiates and maintains vasodilation through a cascade of biological events that culminate in the relaxation of smooth muscle cells that line arteries, veins and lymphatics. Since the early 1980s, an explosion of research in laboratories across the globe has revealed many successes confirming that nitric oxide works within the body's complex biochemistry to help prevent major diseases. Results also validate that it can restore health to those who already suffer from those diseases.

Researchers now know that nitric oxide can significantly reduce high blood pressure and slash the risk of the blood clots that trigger heart attacks and strokes. It can often lower cholesterol levels almost as well as high-priced statin drugs, and it can keep the so-called bad cholesterol from oxidizing into an even nastier artery-clogging form. Nitric oxide can reduce the risk of diabetes and lessens the severity of damage in those who suffer from it. It appears to trigger the pituitary gland into releasing human growth hormone, the same substance shown to slow, and even reverse, the aging process itself. It can also restore erectile function to impotent men, and very likely enhance sexuality for women as well.

In fact, the editors of the highly prestigious journal Science, after voting NO the 1992 Science Molecule of the Year stated, " Nitric oxide helps maintain blood pressure by dilating blood vessels, helps kill foreign invaders in the immune response, is a major mediator of penile erections, and is probably a major biochemical component of long-term memory these are just a few of its benefits."

Nitric oxide (not to be confused with nitrous oxide, otherwise known as the laughing gas your dentist may use as an anesthetic) is a chemical produced in the body that keeps blood vessels dilated, thus increasing blood flow. Nitric oxide also has a wide variety of other benefits, including killing bacteria and viruses and promoting healing of wounds and ulcers. Nitric oxide regulates muscle contraction, signals the long-term adaptive response to exercise, controls nutrient delivery and uptake, widens the blood channels, indirectly initiates fatty-acid oxidation and generates new muscle growth.

Stress, aging, injuries, intense exercise, and fighting disease-causing organisms can all deplete the body of nitric oxide. A human or animal that has insufficient levels of nitric oxide will be unable to perform to the best of its abilities. Nitric oxide synthase (NOS) from which nitric oxide is derived is a pH dependent enzyme. It is active at slightly alkaline conditions but is suppressed by acidic conditions (such as the result of modem American diets) therefore creating a deficiency of nitric oxide. In diabetics, glycolysis and ketoacidosis force pH toward acid conditions and this may account for the reduction of nitric oxide.

Depletion of nitric oxide may be involved in a variety of health problems, including reduced blood flow to the stomach causing stomach ulcers, and in other cases insufficient nitric oxide allows blood pressure to rise excessively in the lungs, causing bleeding. For others, insufficient production of nitric oxide can reduce blood flow to the sex organs, causing impotence. Dr. Jonathan Stamler and his colleagues at Duke University Medical Center showed that nitric oxide binds to hemoglobin, the blood's chemical "magnet" that delivers oxygen to our cells, then carries carbon dioxide back to the lungs for discharging.

What's more, Dr. Stamler and his team convincingly demonstrated that nitric oxide is not just some passive molecular hitch- hiker along for a blood-borne ride. Instead, it serves as the key regulator of blood circulation and lung function. Without nitric oxide, human life would be impossible.

Note: Nitroglycerine was discovered by Alfred Nobel, the man after whom the Noble Prize is named. Nitroglycerine was used as a drug for cardiac treatment for more than 100 years after the accidental discovery that the workers in his nitroglycerine factory had low blood pressure. Through this research the levels of nitric oxide were raised increasing the body's ability to regulate blood pressure. It is now possible to explain the beneficial role of nitric oxide in the treatment of heart disease. The three scientists, Robert F Furchgot, Louis Ignarro, and FeridMurad, won the Nobel Prize in Physiology in 1998 for their pioneering research on nitric oxide.

CHAPTER 2

NO AND PLAQUE PREVENTION

Heart disease. Over six million Americans have it, over 650,000 die from it each year, and countless others worry obsessively about getting it. This worry means stress, and stress may up your odds of developing the condition.

There are many different forms of heart disease. The most common is CAD (coronary artery disease), a condition characterized by coronary vessel blockages that reduce the blood reaching the heart. The second form is hypertensive heart disease. It occurs when the heart itself actually changes in form and function as a result of chronic and untreated high blood pressure.

A study in the journal Circulation revealed that increasing the amount of nitric oxide in the body actually reduced pathological increases in the thickness of plaque-lined vessel walls. Another study published in Circulation showed that nitric oxide improved blood flow in men aged 54-74 who had a history of elevated serum cholesterol and who had shown signs of early coronary artery disease.

*"In the beginner's mind there are many possibilities,
but in the expert's, there are few."*
Shunryu Suzuki

CHAPTER 3

NO MAINTAINS NOT ONLY HEALTHY ARTERIES, BUT VEINS TOO

HOW ATHEROSCLEROSIS HURTS US

Any problems with our arteries or veins that impair our robust, yet also delicate, circulatory system can have disastrous consequences. One of the most common disorders of the circulatory system is *atherosclerosis,* a form of hardening of the lining of the arteries. Almost 5 million people in the U.S. have been diagnosed with atherosclerosis. In this condition, a fatty material called plaque is deposited on the inner layer, or epithelial-cell layer, of the arteries. As the plaque buildup increases over time, it causes a constriction of the arterial volume - the space within the arteries - and this, in turn, restricts blood flow and increases our blood pressure.

Ultimately, atherosclerosis can seriously impair the blood supply to different parts of the body - dramatically so if a piece of plaque breaks off and completely obstructs an artery. If blood supply to the heart is obstructed, a heart attack can occur. If blood supply to a portion of the brain is cut off, a stroke (think of it as a "brain attack") can occur.

Although heart attacks and strokes represent the worst-case scenarios in a circulatory system that is deteriorating, smaller reductions in proper blood flow can rob the body of important nutrients and prevent it from working at its peak form. We consider a certain amount of deterioration of our circulatory system to be a natural part of aging. But, as with most other seemingly inevitable conditions, we can take steps to counteract it.

HOW NITRIC OXIDE PREVENTS ATHEROSCLEROSIS

Several studies have shown that nitric oxide plays a direct role in preventing atherosclerosis. Its action is twofold. First, it acts as a vasodilator, inducing the dilation of arteries in response to certain kinds of stress and other factors. This dilation increases the arterial volume and facilitates blood flow, while lowering blood pressure, the exact opposite of the effects caused by atherosclerotic plaque buildup. Conditions that reduce nitric oxide levels are believed to impair the ability of arteries to dilate properly. Second, nitric oxide decreases the tendency of monocytes (a type of large white blood cells that constitutes roughly 6% of all the body's white blood cells) to adhere to the epithelial cells that line the arteries. What this means, is that nitric oxide can reduce the plaque formation that leads to atherosclerosis, and more

NITRIC OXIDE IMPROVES VENOUS HEALTH

Nitric oxide is an important compound for proper arterial function. In recent years its role in regulating *venous* function as well has become clearer, and several studies have demonstrated its importance in this area. In one study, researchers examined the role of nitric oxide in regulating blood volume in the veins of 24 healthy human subjects, of whom 16 were men and 8 were women. Their ages ranged from 27 to 75 years, with an average age of 50. None had a history of smoking, hypertension, diabetes, or high cholesterol. Furthermore, none had a family history of heart disease.

The study measured venous volume - the space within the veins - by labeling the subjects' blood cells with harmless, low-level radioactive tracers and then measuring the resulting radioactivity in their forearms, where the technique is easy to apply. It was found that they could decrease the venous volume by infusing a compound into the subjects' bloodstream that is known to inhibit the action of a key enzyme in the biochemical pathway for nitric oxide production, i.e., its effect is to reduce nitric oxide. The fact that venous volume decreased in this experiment thus proved that nitric oxide is necessary for maintaining normal levels of blood flow in our veins.

Next, the research team tried infusing a compound that *stimulates* nitric oxide production into the patients' bloodstream, and they found that this *increased* their venous volume. The response was dose-dependent; that is, the increase in venous volume was proportional to the amount of compound administered. This experiment provided further proof of nitric oxide's role in maintaining proper blood flow in our veins as well as our arteries. In their paper, they concluded that "Nitric oxide has an important role in the regulation of venous tone and contributes to resting venous tone in healthy human subjects."

SUPPLEMENTAL ARGININE IS KEY

The many benefits of both nitric oxide and growth hormone can be obtained through arginine. For this reason, arginine is clearly one of the best nutrient bargains currently available. It should be a component in every serious life extender's nutritional program.

Arginine can be found in many foods, including chocolate, wheat germ, wheat flour, buckwheat, granola, oatmeal, dairy products, beef, pork, nuts, seeds, poultry, seafood, chickpeas, and soybeans. However, it is difficult, if not impossible, to obtain high enough levels of arginine from food alone. To obtain the full range of arginine's benefits, supplementation is necessary.

"Sit loosely in the saddle of life."
Robert Louis Stevenson

CHAPTER 4

NO, THE BODY'S SAFE AND NATURAL BLOOD THINNER

You have probably heard that so-called blood thinners are sometimes used to treat heart and hypertensive patients. Blood thinners prevent platelets from becoming sticky and forming clots. The medical term for these thinners is anticoagulants.

One well-known anticoagulant is aspirin. Doctors know that one of aspirin's many properties include the inhibition of platelet clumping. Unfortunately, an anticoagulant like aspirin can have pernicious side effects for many patients, side effects that can range from serious stomach bleeding to kidney damage.

A recent report from the Boston University School of Medicine, cautioned that aspirin could irritate the stomach lining, causing sometimes severe upper gastrointestinal bleeding and hemorrhagic stroke (unchecked bleeding into the brain). So for some patients, "blood thinning" with daily aspirin can be a lifesaver, but for many others it can result in a kind of disease substitution whereby reducing the odds of one bad outcome simply ups the odds of another.

The good news is that researchers have found another "blood thinning" approach that is equally effective in controlling platelets aggregation, but without the side effects like those of aspirin. Drs. M.W. Radomski, R.M.J. Palmer and Salvador Moncada learned that platelets themselves contain their own form of the enzyme, nitric oxide synthase. This ability to form nitric oxide is a "fail-safe" mechanism that limits the capacity of platelets to do inadvertent damage to the blood vessels they are designed to save. Nature has equipped us with our own emergency clot-busters. Not only will nitric oxide prevent your platelets from clotting, it will dilate the blood vessels supplying tissues with a high demand for oxygen and nutrients.

The delivery of oxygen from the lungs to body tissues and the subsequent removal of carbon dioxide waste back to the lungs for exhalation is a complex process. It is largely mediated by hemoglobin, an iron-containing protein found in red blood cells. Recent research has found that hemoglobin also binds to a third gas, nitric oxide. This is ferried along with oxygen and carbon dioxide and can be released when needed to dilate arterial vessels, thereby allowing more blood flow to tissues, which require extra oxygen.

To reiterate, nitric oxide figures prominently as a kind of fail-safe mechanism for blood platelets, which are, by the way, the body's smallest cells. When a vessel sustains an injury, platelets become 'sticky' and aggregate into clots that serve as miniature dams to stanch further blood loss. This protective mechanism can sometimes go awry in patients whose arteries have undergone narrowing and occlusion due to atherosclerotic plaque. Large blood clots can be deadly, especially when they occur in vital areas like the coronary arteries or the arteries that feed the brain. To prevent this outcome, heart patients are often prescribed anticoagulants to inhibit platelet stickiness.

Unfortunately, many of the conventional "blood thinners," including aspirin, can trigger other side effects, from stomach ulcers to hemorrhagic stroke. Nitric oxide will help open arteries and reduce the stickiness of platelets.

"Is it not strange that desire should so many years outlive performance?"
William Shakespeare

CHAPTER 5

JUST SAY NO TO SEXUAL DYSFUNCTION AND SAY YES TO SEXUAL ENHANCEMENT

During the early 1990's, urologist Dr. Jacob Raijfer and other researchers at UCLA discovered that in the healthy penis, blood inflow is triggered when nerve endings release the short-lived gas nitric oxide. This is the same nitric oxide that had so recently emerged as the chief natural relaxant for the smooth muscle rings in arteries themselves. The researchers determined that nitric oxide, like a tipped domino, initiates a series of biochemical reactions in the penis that ultimately engorge it with blood and allow it to remain erect.

When declaring nitric oxide the 1992 Molecule of the Year, the editors of Science referred to the pivotal discoveries at UCLA when they wrote, "This year scientists proved definitively that in men, nitric oxide translates sexual excitement into potency by causing erections. The pelvic nerves get a message from the brain and make nitric oxide in response. Nitric oxide dilates the blood vessels throughout the crucial areas of the penis, blood rushes in, and the penis rises to the occasion."

In a report in The New England Journal of Medicine, Dr. Raijfer and his colleagues suggested that defects in the nitric oxide system may prevent sufficient inflow of blood or, alternatively, may cause blood to leak out prematurely, in either case quashing an erection. Dr. Raijfer stated that up to 81 percent of impotence in American men was directly attributable to some form of nitric oxide failure.

Recently, researchers have discovered that it's not just men who undergo changes in their sex-organ blood-flow patterns. Women endure nearly identical changes as well. To be sure, blood engorgement of the vaginal tissues may be harder to see than the changes in a penis as it becomes erect, but more and more doctors now believe that a healthy sexual response in women is as dependent on a well-functioning vasculature as it is in men. Vaginal lubrication, for instance, is just one example of a process that's highly dependent on ample blood flow in the urogenital arteries. Nitric oxide will definitely enhance blood- flow patterns to the female sex organ.

Below are the "Seven Steps to Erection" in terms of the biochemical pathway:

1. Sexual stimulation causes a variety of nerves originating in the brain to start firing.

2. Once stimulated, these nerves cause the release of the neurotransmitter acetylcholine in the penis.

3. This acetylcholine, in turn, causes the endothelial cells in penile arteries to begin producing nitric oxide. (Endothelial cells are small cells that make up capillaries and line every blood vessel and lymph duct in the body.)

4. Nitric oxide then triggers the release of another naturally occurring chemical called cyclic guanosine monophosphate (GMP). Cyclic GMP is one of the any potent vasodilating chemicals found in the human body.

5. As cyclic GMP levels build, the smooth muscles of the penile arteries relax, the vessels dilate, and increased blood flow causes swelling of the corpus cavemosa, producing an erection.

6. Even as nitric oxide continues to build up cyclic GMP, an enzyme   begins to break it down. This enzyme, phosphodiesterase, appears to act as a brake on the overall system, preventing erections from becoming excessive or permanent.

7. Following climax or other cessation of the sexual stimulation, the penile nerves stop firing and the nerve endings cease releasing acetylcholine. Without the acetylcholine signal, the endothelial cells cut back on nitric oxide production. What little cyclic GMP remains free floating is soon broken down by phosphodiesterase. The smooth muscles of the penis blood vessels once again contract, and the penis goes into its non-arousal, compact state.

A well-advertised pharmaceutical drug for sexual enhancement works by an entirely different mechanism. This drug blocks the enzyme, phosphodiesterase. Without this enzyme to put the brakes on cyclic GMP, levels of this potent vasodilator can create potential problems.

CHAPTER 6

HOW NO CAN HELP DIABETICS

Diabetes mellitus is the seventh leading cause of death in the United States, killing over 60,000 people every year. People with varying forms of diabetes all share the inability to keep their blood-sugar levels from rising to dangerous levels. Such elevation, in tum, can lead to progressive damage to the heart, large blood vessels, capillaries, kidneys, nervous system and brain. The body's natural vasodilator is nitric oxide, but its production by diabetics is often 50 percent or more below normal levels. In addition, any nitric oxide that is formed is very tightly bound to hemoglobin within red blood cells (and possibly to other heme proteins in other cells) so that it cannot be easily released to cause a needed increase in blood flow. Adequate oxygen is necessary for the activity of nitric oxide synthase (NOS), an enzyme that generates nitric oxide from L-arginine combined with L-Citrulline. Circulation is impaired in diabetics and people with heart conditions that limit available NOS and nitric oxide.

Diabetes also promotes atherosclerosis and can trigger life-threatening seizures caused by low blood pH, when the blood becomes too acidic. Poor circulation in the extremities predisposes many diabetic men to impotence. In men and women alike, diabetes can result in gangrene in the hands and feet, a catastrophic infection that can require amputation of the affected limbs. Diabetics can also become blind due to damage to blood vessels in the eyes.

When blood serum levels climb high and stay that way too long, they set off a number of harmful biochemical reactions in the blood. Excess sugar, for instance, can bind to hemoglobin, a damaging process known as glycosylation. Glucose can also react with certain proteins in the blood, producing mega molecules that can destroy fragile capillaries and reduce a diabetic's life span by as much as one-third.

Diabetes also accelerates hardening of the arteries in many patients. One likely contributor to this is "lipid peroxidation," when blood fats such as LCD are turned rancid by oxygen free radicals. Nitric oxide can reduce lipid peroxidation. In one study, thirty patients with diabetes mellitus had their nitric oxide increased and after three months they had a significant decrease in lipid peroxidation - a major benefit in the fight against atherosclerosis. Dr. Ian I. Joffe from Beth Deaconess Medical Center in Boston concluded from this study that cardiac dysfunction in diabetes mellitus is due to impaired availability of nitric oxide.

Nitric oxide may have an even more direct benefit, especially for those suffering the adult-onset form of diabetes. Researchers at the Medical College of Wisconsin have demonstrated that nitric oxide production can restore blood vessel function and improve other pathological changes caused by diabetes.

CHAPTER 7

NO AND NEUROTRANSMISSION

Diabetic patients are particularly at risk of damage to sensory and motor nerves in the feet or to dysfunction of the autonomic nervous system that innervates internal organs, for example, the intestines. The clinical diagnosis of the latter condition is gastroparesis. Nitric oxide is an important signaling molecule conveying information from one nerve to another, including non-cholinergic, non-adrenergic, (NCNA) nerves. NCNA nerves control smooth muscle cells, which regulate gastric emptying and intestinal motility. Reduced availability of nitric oxide in diabetic patients may be one of the causes of gastroparesis.

Nerves communicate with one another across synapses and several biochemical compounds diffuse from one nerve to the second nerve. Nitric oxide is one of these biochemical "neuro-transmitter" molecules and is produced by both brain tissue and peripheral nerves.

Nitric oxide has both a direct and indirect effect on neuro-transmission. The direct effect relates to permeability of nerve membranes regulating ion transport that is important for nerve signal transmission. Indirectly, nitric oxide enables nerves to properly function by causing increase in blood flow (vasodilatation) allowing essential oxygen and nutrients to be transported to nerve cells.

Nitric oxide, by affecting cyclic GMP, allows phosphorylation (addition of a phosphate group) of ion channels, especially potassium channels necessary for normal transmission of nerve signals. Nitric oxide also increases blood flow. This allows sufficient oxygen and glucose to be transported to nerve cells, positively affecting ATP (adenosine triphosphate) production, our primary energy source, and in turn, facilitates potassium/ sodium homeostasis essential for neurotransmission. Increases in blood flow may also allow the oxygen dependent isoform, iNOS, to produce more nitric oxide. (iNOS is a form of NO that helps in synaptic transmission, the process of nervous information from nerve to nerve across gaps (synapses) and from peripheral nerves to the brain.)

In summary, nitric oxide may reduce pain associated with diabetes directly by increasing cyclic GMP, indirectly by increasing circulation to restore normal membrane potential and reduce pressure on nerves due to localized edema.

CHAPTER 8

NO: THE NATURAL WAY to LOWER HIGH BLOOD PRESSURE

Over sixty million Americans suffer from hypertension, otherwise known as high blood pressure. Untold others are heading along in their footsteps. Often referred to as the "silent killer," the disorder so rarely announces itself with any warning sign. Hypertension is one of the leading causes of illness, disability, and death in the United States. Left untreated, chronic elevation of blood pressure nearly triples your risk of all the major circulatory disorders, from heart failure to peripheral artery disease. It accelerates the hardening of the arteries, damages your heart by enlarging one or more of its chambers, increases the risk of blood clots that can trigger heart attacks and strokes, and can even lead to a rupture of blood vessels in your brain, causing the so-called hemorrhagic stroke.

Researchers for the National Institutes of Health in Washington, D.C., found that African Americans are particularly vulnerable to hypertension due to a reduced sensitivity of blood vessels to nitric oxide.

All women tend to enter their adulthood with lower blood pressure than men, but by middle age they tend to catch up, and often exceed blood-pressure levels in males of the same age.

24

Blood pressure is relatively easy to understand. With each contraction of the powerful left chamber of your heart, oxygen-rich blood is propelled forward into your aorta, the body's largest artery. From here, the blood flow divides to other arteries, which in turn, branch off into progressively smaller arteries, and eventually tiny arterioles and capillaries. This path from heart, to aorta, arterioles, and capillaries, is the expeditious transportation of blood to every organ and tissue in your body.

So, how does your circulatory system accomplish this amazingly complex logistical task? It does this, by selectively dilating the "pipes" that carry blood to high-demand regions while constricting those that supply regions that are lower on the priority list. Doctors refer to these two complementary mechanisms as vasodilation and vasoconstriction. Your arterial system accomplishes this opening and narrowing via the action of smooth muscle rings that wrap around arterial " pipes" themselves.

Operating properly, the smooth muscle action is a miraculous example of biochemical orchestration, with the principal conductor being nitric oxide. Researchers are now realizing that nitric oxide created by the endothelial cells lining your arteries, is really the principal blood pressure regulator of the body.

Once produced and released by the endothelium, nitric oxide causes the arterial smooth muscles making up the vessel walls to relax enlarging the interior diameter of the artery, and ultimately letting more blood flow through.

It has only recently been discovered that damage from the standard coronary heart disease risk factors, from hypertension to high cholesterol, impairs the ability of your endothelium to produce nitric oxide when and where it is needed.

CHAPTER 9

NO AND THE IMMUNE SYSTEM

A healthy, well-functioning immune system is a marvel of natural microbiology, physics and biochemistry. Without it, we could not survive for even the shortest period of time on this planet. Every living organism, from animals to plants, has an immune system, each with differences that promote individual survival and health.

Besides physical, mechanical and chemical means of preventing microorganisms from entering our body, innate immunity also has cellular defenses. This next line of defense consists of specialized immune cells that destroy the invader once it has entered our body. We have natural killer (NK) cells that hunt down and destroy virus-infected cells and cancer cells, as well as cells infected with bacteria and protozoa. Also, there are a variety of phagocytes, called "cell-eaters", including the macro- phages that filter and remove debris from the blood and make up an important part of the first line of defense strategy of the immune system in eliminating bacteria and parasites.

Recent research believes that small bursts of nitric oxide fired by macrophage combat our "enemies" in at least two distinctive ways. First nitric oxide interferes with iron containing molecules crucial to cellular respiration. This kills the "enemy" by poisoning it. Among the common infections that nitric oxide is known to kill by this mechanism:

- Salmonella - a bacteria that causes food poisoning
- Candida albicans - a common form of yeast infection
- E. coli 0157 - the infamous bacterial killer
- Chlamydia - a widespread, sexually transmitted disease
- Helicobacter pylori - a bacteria that been linked to causing, peptic ulcer, migraines and heart disease

Secondly, nitric oxide provides a mechanism to neutralize infectious invaders and possible tumor cells. It appears to have the ability to interfere with the enzymes necessary for DNA replication in harmful organisms. Nitric oxide can therefore keep infectious agents and cancer cells from reproducing.

Research on nitric oxide's effect on cancer has become a priority for many scientists. The Virulence Journal, (2012) reported a study that showed that increasing the amount of nitric oxide would inhibit tumor growth. Numerous studies have examined the effect of nitric oxide on a spectrum of different cancers in vivo and in vitro and in many cases, nitric oxide seems to hold considerable promise as an adjunct to traditional care.

One area of clinical practice where nitric oxide is playing an increasingly important role is wound healing. From helping patients overcome trauma more quickly to expediting recovery after surgery, many doctors have realized that nitric oxide helps boost the body's innate restorative powers.

Scientists studying wounds have long observed that the affected tissues often have low levels of nitric oxide in them. Dr. Adrian Barbul, in the Journal of Surgical Research, found that more nitric oxide reduced inflammation and sped up the rate of healing. The latest research has also shown that macrophages can use nitric oxide to poison the internal metabolism of enemy cells, or to interfere with the ability of these adversaries to reproduce their DNA. Nitric oxide is now known to be an effective killer of a wide variety of common infectious disease agents, from Salmonella to Chlamydia. Nitric oxide fired by macrophages and other immune cells also have the power to destroy some tumors.

CHAPTER 10

NO'S EFFECT ON OTHER CONDITIONS

Throughout this booklet, I have informed you about the ways nitric oxide can benefit your body's most critical physio- logical systems. From tuning up your heart and cardio vasculature to providing your immune system with the necessary firepower to combat infections, nitric oxide is emerging as one of human-kind's most beneficial ally.

Nitric oxide will help to treat many of the harmful underlying disorders, like high blood pressure, that have for so long put a burden on your body's crucial blood-filtering organs. Perhaps even more promising is the possibility that nitric oxide can help prevent kidney disease long before it has a chance to develop. If your kidneys are not now diseased, increasing your nitric oxide today may well help inoculate you against future problems. In the rest of this section, I will be examining some of the many other disorders for, which nitric oxide is very beneficial. As Dr. Jonathan S. Stamler of Duke University stated, "Nitric oxide does everything, everywhere. You cannot name a major cellular response or physiological effect in which nitric oxide is not implicated today".

NO AND THE BRAIN

The healthy brain consumes twenty-five percent of the body's oxygen supply and an astonishing seventy percent of its blood glucose. It also produces an array of chemicals. Cut off blood supply for more than a few minutes, and brain cells quickly begin to die. If blood flow is just slightly reduced, the resulting reduction in oxygen on a chronic basis can contribute to a spectrum of mental disorders, from impaired thinking to disorders of senility.

Just as nitric oxide plays a key role in relaxing coronary arteries to guarantee a plentiful blood supply to your heart, so does this mechanism now appear to regulate blood flow to your brain. A 1993 study in Brain Research showed that inhibiting the enzyme used to make nitric oxide caused constriction of the arteries supplying the brain. The body responded by elevating blood pressure to make sure enough blood still made it through. When the researchers increased the amount of nitric oxide the vessels dilated and blood pressure normalized.

Nitric oxide has other functions in the brain, besides orchestrating blood flow. The way different nerve cells "communicate" with one another is through the release of specific messenger chemicals called neurotransmitters. These are typically secreted in the synapse (the tiny gap that separates the end of one nerve cell from another). Serotonin, dopamine, and noradrenaline are just three of the more popularly known neuro- transmitters. Recently, neuroscientists have learned that nitric oxide functions also as a neurotransmitter, facilitating communication among nerve cells whether they are connected via synapses or not.

According to researchers at Stanford University School of Medicine, nitric oxide may well be the " key" for long-term memory. In fact, they were able to show that by inhibiting the enzyme that makes nitric oxide in the brain long-term memory storage was compromised.

Other brain researchers have begun to examine the role of nitric oxide in diseases such as Alzheimer's and Parkinson's. In patients suffering either of these disorders, there is frequently a significant reduction in the nitric oxide being produced in their brain. Recent articles in both Nature (Dec. 2013) and the Journal of Neurological Sciences (April 2005) offered evidence that this reduction may hamper memory storage and reduce blood flow to the brain. The latter may at once contribute to and be exacerbated by a deposit of a specific kind of plaque, called beta-amyloid, that is a hallmark of several degenerative brain diseases including Alzheimer's. This plaque, though chemically different from the atherosclerotic plaque that clogs heart arteries, seems equally damaging to endothelial cells in the small cerebral blood vessels. Restoring healthy levels of nitric oxide in the brain enhances its ability to function at its peak.

NO AND THE AGING PROCESS

In recent years, researchers have focused attention on a key hormone produced by the pituitary gland and known as HGH (human growth hormone). When we are young, HGH directs much of the growth process. It oversees tissue repair throughout the body. As we get older HGH production begins to reduce. By the age of fifty, the pituitary gland of many people releases only very slight amounts. By old age, fully half or more of adults are partially to totally deficient in HGH release. Scientists at the University of California at San Francisco did a study on whether nitric oxide is capable of increasing HGH in adults. The results showed there was a six-fold rise in HGH.

What is certain is that nitric oxide can benefit one of the most important age-related physiological declines: the damage to blood vessels, which itself serves as the first tilted domino in so many deleterious chain reactions.

NO AND PREGNANT WOMEN

There is a unique form of hypertension called preeclampsia that affects an estimated nine to twelve percent of pregnant women, usually but not always during a first pregnancy. Symptoms generally develop in the final trimester and usually feature dangerously elevated blood pressure, fluid retention that leads to swollen hands and feet and a puffy face, and elevated levels of protein in the urine. In severe cases, the condition can evolve into life-threatening eclampsia itself. In the United States, Great Britain, and Scandinavia, eclampsia is the leading cause of death for mothers and infants alike in the moments immediately after childbirth.

What triggers preeclampsia remains mysterious, but clues now point to a failure of nitric oxide production. In 1991, researchers from the University of Cincinnati College of Medicine showed that the placenta could generate nitric oxide that then acts to dilate the blood vessels of the fetus, thus promoting an adequate blood supply. A recent article in the American Journal of Obstetrics and Gynecology reported that nitric oxide seems to inhibit "spontaneous" contractions of the uterus and a woman 's risk of delivering her child early.

NO AND THE LUNGS

Scientists have discovered a major new function for the blood protein called hemoglobin. In addition to delivering oxygen (0) to the body's tissues and removing carbon dioxide (CO), it delivers a gas called nitric oxide (NO), which has important roles like regulating blood pressure.

Asthma refers to a group of related diseases caused by constriction of the breathing passages of the lung. Fluid then frequently accumulates in the little terminal bronchial sacs' leading to inflammation and a further reduction in a victim 's ability to take in a refreshing breath of air. Researchers at the National Heart and Lung Institute in England showed that the mechanisms that keep bronchial passages open in the lungs is controlled entirely by nitric oxide.

Increasing nitric oxide available to the lungs via inhalers has become an accepted therapy for a number of more severe lung-related diseases, including adult respiratory distress syndrome, pulmonary hypertension, and chronic obstructive pulmonary disease (COPD, which is the fourth leading cause of death in the U.S.).

NO AND WOUND HEALING

Nitric oxide and its interrelationship with essential growth factors is critically involved in the entire continuum of events associated with wound repair, including cell division, maturation, neovascularization, and collagen synthesis including proper cross-linking of collagen fibers.

Nitric oxide is a powerful stimulator of cell division. This is called proliferation, one cell into two, four into eight, and so on. For wounds to heal, new tissue is formed through induced division of existing cells. Several of the 10-20 known growth factors are necessary to induce cell division required in tissue repair. Of these, epidermal growth factor and/or keratinocyte growth factor, which are important for re-epithelialization and wound closure, cannot perform their biological function without nitric oxide as a common chemical mediator. It is also important in duplicating some of the components of the cell so that each new cell is identical to its parent.

Without cell division and receptor formation, mediated in part by NO, wound healing will not occur. Formation of new blood vessels, called angiogenesis, is essential for wound healing otherwise newly formed tissue will eventually deteriorate again due to lack of oxygen and nutrients. Growth factors, including vascular endothelial growth factor determines the extent of revascularization of damaged tissues. All growth factors bind to receptors on the cell surface and generate nitric oxide-mediated cyclic GMP. Therefore, nitric oxide is a powerful and necessary mediator of angiogenesis.

NO AND EYE HEALTH

Nitric Oxide may also be a critical regulator of ocular blood flow and neurotransmission. Recent studies are describing the essential role that NO plays in the eyes, and, particularly in the choroid, retina, and optic nerve. Various eye disorders, such as diabetic retinopathy, glaucoma, and age-related macular degeneration (ARMD), can be correlated with a NO deficiency.

Nitric oxide produced in the eyes regulates ocular circulation both inside and outside the eyeball. NO produced in the capillaries of the retina causes them to respond efficiently to changes in blood pressure and oxygen levels. The importance of ocular blood flow is demonstrated in diabetic retinopathy where reduced blood flow and capillary damage result in hypoxia and edema in the retina, eventually causing vision loss. Not surprisingly, the underlying mechanism is endothelial dysfunction, a process defined as the loss of NO production or availability.

In terms of macular degeneration, low NO levels lead to decline in neural and endothelial control of circulation to the choroid of the eye, which is critical for central visual function. ARMD eyes likewise demonstrate a decrease in retinal NO with neuronal degeneration.

NO Regulates Intraocular Pressure

Inside the eye, fluid called the aqueous or vitreous humor (depending on whether it's in front of or behind the lens) provides the pressure needed to hold the eye's shape. The amount of aqueous fluid and its flow in the front of the eye determine whether intraocular pressures go up or down, so several mechanisms regulate the fluid's volume by making sure that the amount of fluid released in the front of the eye is offset by allowing drainage. One of these mechanisms is the trabecular meshwork.

The trabecular meshwork is like a one-way valve that opens to let aqueous humor circulate and drain in the front of the eye. When the meshwork fails--which can be due to normal cells, DNA damage or other causes--fluid can't ci intraocular pressure builds, and glaucoma develoḷ

So how does all of this relate to nitric oxide? It turns out that the trabecular meshwork is regulated by cells that depend in part on nitric oxide. Glaucoma treatments work by lowering intraocular pressure, but none of the current medications affect the trabecular meshwork directly. That may be about to change. After many years of trial-and-error, researchers have finally realized that increasing nitric oxide in our body, helps target the trabecular meshwork.

Restoring NO availability improves blood flow, supports normal intraocular pressure, and is neuroprotective in the eye. Thus, considering NO supplementation if you have any of these devastating eye disorders is of vital importance.

"The body is the soul's house. Shouldn't we therefore take care of our house so that it doesn't fall into ruin?"
Philo Judaeus

CHAPTER 11

NO FOR FITNESS AND STRENGTH TRAINING

Nitric Oxide (NO) scientifically known as L-arginine, has become a very popular product in the sports nutrition industry. Nitric Oxide increases blood flow to the muscles which in turn, helps to deliver and transport blood and nutrients more adequately to these working muscles.

During physical activity, there's an increase in cardiac output and blood flow redistribution to muscle fibers. As we exercise, muscles become oxygen-depleted. In the absence, of oxygen, the body begins to produce lactic acid which will eventually lead to muscle fatigue, to the extent that we can exercise no more. NO reduces the amount of lactic acid produced during exercise and extends the amount of time until exhaustion. By speeding up the delivery of oxygen and nutrients to the muscles under stress, NO improves their response to exercise and so increases sports performance. It is also known to speed up the removal of the exercise generated ammonia and increase glucose uptake by cells.

A recent study showed that L-arginine's role in reducing exercise induced increase in plasma lactate and ammonia. Extended time until muscle failure. Taken together with BCAAs and glutamine, arginine can improve training efficiency by increasing blood oxygen carrying capacity.

Another interesting fact about NO, is that nitric oxide acts to reduce inflammation. This should be of great interest to bodybuilders as it has the potential to reduce pain associated with subjecting muscles to extreme stress. It has also been reported that NO may affect the release of adrenaline from the adrenal medulla.

Perhaps one of the most important effects of arginine supplementation for bodybuilders and all athletes is its ability to stimulate growth hormone production. Scientific research shows that resting growth hormone levels increases with oral ingestion of L-arginine combined with exercise.

Nitric oxide supplements are very popular among athletes and bodybuilders, they promote vasodilation and help the body to deliver precious nutrients to the muscles cells and so improve performance. Gym goers love to feel the pumping effect given by NO supplements.

L-arginine and L-citrulline are two effective ingredients in increasing nitric oxide production and can, at times, deliver other benefits that directly impact muscle growth. Also, taking a good Vitamin B-complex, can help lower homocysteine. High amounts of homocysteine in the blood, blocks activity of eNOS (endothelial nitric oxide synthase).

Homocysteine is an amino acid that is produced in the body. High homocysteine levels in the blood can damage the lining of the arteries. Also, high homocysteine levels may make blood clots more easily than it should. Most people who have a high homocysteine level don't get enough folate (folic acid), vitamin B6 or vitamin B12 in their diet.

Polyphenols, micronutrients that we get through certain plant-based foods (berries, apples, grapes, cherries, beans), stimulates eNOS. By acting as scavengers of free radical damage, polyphenols may prevent these radicals from interacting with and destroying nitric oxide.

FREQUENTLY ASKED QUESTIONS

ABOUT NO

We asked one manufacturer of a supplement that supports the production of nitric oxide to answer these questions.

How Does NO Work?

Nitric oxide (NO), produced in the endothelium, signals the smooth muscle, which makes up most of the blood vessel, to dilate (relax). It also prevents plaque from forming on the endothelium and keeps the blood cells from clumping. Many vascular diseases may be caused by a nitric oxide deficiency.

How can I maintain a healthy level of NO?

The active ingredient of L-Arginine, a precursor used by the body to produce nitric oxide, helps to widen blood vessels so blood can flow efficiently to the heart.

I am at a high risk for heart disease, what can I do?

Because of its usefulness in checking hypertension, I believe NO is an ideal preventative measure for presently healthy individuals at risk for heart disease who hope to safeguard their heart and prevent long-term pathological changes such as congestive heart failure.

I've read that menopause can cause women to suffer from vaginal dryness. Will an NO supplement help me?

NO for women would be an excellent suggestion. Nitric oxide synthesis can help the sexual functions of females, including enhanced lubrication and sensitivity, as well as sexual response.

How do I take NO supplements?

The products must be taken when the stomach is as empty as possible, especially for the first month. Stop eating for one hour before and one hour after taking the product. This is essential to insure rapid absorption of the ingredients in order to produce the desired effects.

Can I take these products with my medication or other supplements?

Anti-inflammatory drugs and certain herbs block formation of nitric oxide. They prevent NO products from working. All anti-inflammatory drugs and all other anti-inflammatory supplements need to be stopped for at least the first four weeks while taking NO products.

I am a Type 2 diabetic. Which of your products will benefit me?

NO supplementation is essential to maintaining a diabetic's wellbeing. Key nutrients coupled with nitric oxide precursor technology help maintain proper circulation to the extremities and internal organs. Supplementation will support the production of nitric oxide and is appropriate where increased blood flow is indicated and beneficial.

I have difficulty maintaining an erection and I don't want to take drugs. Is there a natural solution?

Over half of the males over forty suffer from erectile dysfunction. Some men lack certain nutrients, which nitric oxide quickly and effectively replaces. L-Arginine increases nitric oxide production and nitric oxide increases blood flow to the genitalia, which enhances perceived firmness of erection.

Are there any side effects taking NO supplements?

The most common nitric oxide supplement side effects are primarily minor and include nausea, diarrhea, headaches and stomach problems. Always consult with a doctor before using any nitric oxide supplement as there are dangerous interactions with medications that can occur. Antihypertensive drugs combined with arginine, might cause blood pressure to drop dangerously low levels. Also avoid taking nitric oxide supplements with nitrates or other medication which increase blood flow to the heart. This might cause increased dizziness and lightheadedness.

TESTIMONIALS

"In recent studies with cardiovascular and diabetic patients, we have concluded that they have a low amount of nitric oxide production. I highly recommend a good NO product."

Chris Greene D.C., Atlanta, GA

"I have been taking an excellent NO supplement for several months and I find it to be very useful and very effective. I enjoy taking the product because I am able to feel how it affects my body in different ways, primarily in sexual stimulation and muscle enhancement. I also take it when I work out and have really noticed a difference in that area as well."

Roger Gunderson, MHsc, Ph.D., ND, Camarillo, CA

"I used to get a sharp pain in my right leg that caused quite a bit of discomfort. I started taking a NO supplement and within a few days the pain went away and hasn't been back."

Selma Schefler, San Diego, CA

"My name is Guillermo Leon and I am 57 years old. I am a diabetic and also have heart disease. I use to go to the gym every morning for moderate exercise but all I felt like doing was to stay in bed. I had numbness in both legs; there was little or no sensation in my feet or toes, constant headaches and my chest would hurt from the angioplasty procedure performed several years ago I didn't feel very alive, all my energy was gone out of my body and even my youngest grandchild noticed my weak   and feeble appearance.

" My son brought me a supply of a great NO supplement ... it's been the best thing that has happened to me. I feel rejuvenated with lots of energy to go to the gym and walk along the beach with my grandchildren. I now have a lust for living again, I am able to jump and run and play in the park with all seven of my grandchildren. My headaches are almost completely vanished and the dull pain in my chest has actually gone away. I am now able to get rest and sleep since taking NO, I would recommend this product to anyone with diabetes and/or heart disease."

Guillermo Leon, San Diego, CA

"My boyfriend and I am started taking a great NO supplement. For the time we have been taking these supplements (about three weeks), we have taken our sexual intimacy to a higher level. I am VERY impressed with how these products are working. I would highly recommend to any couples to try taking NO supplements."

MaryRose Phillips, Amarillo, TX

"I have suffered with progressive Diabetic Neuropathy for several years. The neuropathy had gotten to the point that I had lost feeling in my feet, legs and hands.   After taking a NO supplement for a couple of weeks, I noticed that feelings in my feet, legs and hands had returned, my coordination improved and the shooting pains in my legs subsided. What a wonderful product! I am very appreciative knowing that NO has helped my quality of life."

Joseph F. Harrison, San Diego, CA

"Being 42 years old, each year seems to be much tougher to stay in optimum health. I have always lived a very active physical life and with that came injuries. Since having seven surgeries from slipped disc to dislocated shoulder, it has been a bit challenging keeping my body in shape. Until now!

I have been taking a great NO supplement for two months and have seen results that I have not seen prior with other products. For example, at the gym, I increased my weights by 10 percent during the second week of taking NO and by the fourth week, I increased my weights another 10 percent, totaling 20 percent. I now ride my bike 100 miles a week. Overall, I have lost five pounds and added more muscle mass. I am very impressed with this product and believe it has a great potential to serve the health industry in so many ways."

Howard Lim, Los Angeles, CA

"My family has a history of heart challenges, and I unfortunately inherited those same traits. NO has become a regular part of my daily routine. My doctor and I were amazed when we saw my last blood test. Now I won 't go a day without my NO supplement."

Annette Wilson, Albuquerque, NM

"I am 54 years old and was recently diagnosed with erectile dysfunction. This has affected me physically and emotionally. Last month a friend of mine introduced me to a supplement of NO. Since taking this product on a daily basis, there has been a change in me not only physically, also emotionally. I have more confidence; my self-esteem has risen and my outlook on life has gotten better. Thank you, thank you!"

Brian Lawrence, New York, NY

"I am 70 years old and in good health. It is my pleasure to share my experience with a product that has had such a positive impact on me and the people with whom I have shared this information.

I have always been physical and athletic, but not so much at age 70. It is important that I keep my body in good shape and I am told I am still looking like the age of 45. In my effort to stay in shape, I went to a trainer, who I swear must be a Marine Corps drill sergeant. After my first session, I threatened to call the police and file charges for attempted murder. I thought to use NO supplement, and I was never sour again after regular usage of this product. I also take it when I do strenuous physical activities or need extra energy. I had several nagging health issues from the lack of circulation. My extremities were always cold. I had to sleep with socks on my feet at night even when it was not winter. My hands stayed cold to the touch. I would also suffer from gout when I ate seafood. I noticed that when taking my NO supplement, I had fewer problems.

My wife suffered from nightly leg and feet cramps to the extent that she would have to get out of bed in the middle of the night to get relief. After taking a NO product, neither she nor I have that problem. Two friends of mine had cancer and after taking the product, they are having favorable recovery. Before taking the product, one was having surgery every year to remove reoccurring cancer growth. That is no longer the case.

A man's sexual "fountain of youth" is NO. It is great at the age of 70, I can feel the excitement and rigidity of age 18 again. The only disadvantage of the product is that your partner does not get much sleep any more. In my profession as a Pastor and Counselor, I often encounter many people who are sexually dysfunctional. It is a serious problem to their relation- ship and threatens the union often, sometimes ending in divorce because of the problem. Therefore, when I find a product that produces such excellent and exciting results, I can help families be more functional and stay together. These products could be called wonder products because they address so many ailments giving people health and happiness.

Pastor Robert L. Chew, Ph.D., Zion Hill Church, Rodeo, CA

CONCLUSION

Nitric oxide is such a ubiquitous and important substance in the human body that at least one top researcher has stated, "It does everything, everywhere!" Indeed, a host of seemingly unrelated miscellaneous health problems, from Alzheimer's to diabetes, all seem to have one thing in common: they are caused or exacerbated by a deficiency of nitric oxide.

Researchers searching for ways to treat and prevent these disorders have begun to investigate a way to boost nitric oxide levels and benefit patients. Such benefits can occur through several different processes that nitric oxide regulates. Nitric oxide-mediated dilation of blood vessels keeps oxygen and glucose flowing freely to the brain, thus preventing the cognitive decline that hypoxia can cause. Nitric oxide also serves as a neuro-transmitter that allows nerve cells to communicate even when they are not directly connected.

Among other effects, nitric oxide may also promote the release of insulin, which could benefit diabetics, and human growth hormone (HGH), which improves body composition and may play a role in retarding the aging process.

REFERENCES

Baechle, T., Earle, Essentials of Strength Training and Conditioning, NSCA 2000

Barbul, A., "IV Alimentation with High NO Levels Improve Wound Healing and Immune Function," *Journal of Surgical Research* 38 (1985)

Blakeslee, S., "Surprise Discovery in Blood," *The New York Times,* March 21, 1996, Al-A22

Bokelman, T., "NO Augments Abnormal Endothelium- Dependent Skeletal Muscle Vasodilation in Patients with Coronary Artery Disease," *Circulation,* Supplement I, 92 (1995) R. Essentials of

Buchanan, J.E., "The Role of NO in the Regulation of Cerebral Blood Flow," *Brain Research,* 610 (1993)

Cardillo,C., "Racial Differences in NO," *Hypertension* 31 (1998) DeGroote, M.A., "Genetic and Redox Determines of NO," *Proceedings of the National Academy of Sciences* 92 (1995)

Green, S.J., "Antimicrobial and Immunopathologic Effects of Cytokine-Induced NO," *Current Opinion in Infectious Diseases* 6 (1993)

Joffe, I.I., " Impaired NO Availability Contributes to the Cardiac Dysfunction of Diabetes," *Circulation* (abstracts), 96 (1997)

Kelly, J.P., "Risk of Aspirin-Associated Major Upper G.I. Bleeding," *The Lancet* 348 (1996)

Kharitonov, S.A., " Acute and Chronic Effects of Cigarette Smoking on Exhaled NO," *American Journal of Respiratory and Critical Care Medicine,* 152 (1995)

Koshland, D.E., "The Molecule of The Year," *Science* 258 (1992)

Kuiper, M.A., "Decreased Cerebrospinal Fluid Nitrate Levels in Parkinson's Disease and Multiple Atrophy Patients," *Journal of Neurological Sciences,* 121 (1994)

Mol Cell Biochem Aug 2004; 23(6):403-7
Myatt, L., " The Action of NO in the Perfused Human Fetal- Placental Circulation," *American Journal of Obstetrics and Gynecology,* 164 (1991)

Pieper, G.M., " NO Pathway in Diabetes," *Journal of Cardio- vascular Pharmacology* 25 (1995)

Peiper, **H., *Natural Solutions for Sexual Enhancement,***
Safe Goods Publishing, 1996

Peiper, **H., *The Secrets of Staying Young,*** Safe Goods Publishing, 1994
Radomski, **M.W., "NO** Pathways," *Proceedings of the National Academy of Sciences* 87 (1990)

Raijfer, **J., "NO** as a Mediator of Relaxation of the Corpus Cavemosum," *The New England Journal of Urology* 326 (1992)

Schuman, E.M, "A Requirement for the Intercellular Messenger Nitric Oxide Long-Term Potentiation, " *Science,* 254 (1991)

Stamler,J., "Blood Flow Regulation by S-Nitrosohemoglobin In the Physiological Oxygen Gradient," *Science, 276* (1997)

Takeda, Y., " Inhibitory Effect of NO on Growth of Rat Mammary Tumors," *Cancer Research* 35 (1975)

Thomas T., "Beta-Amyloid Vasoactivity and Vascular Endothelial Damage," *Nature,* 380 (1996)

AUTHOR'S BIOGRAPHY

Dr. Howard Peiper is a Doctor of Naturopathic Medicine. In 1972, he received his degree in Naturopathy. After a decade in private practice, Dr. Peiper became a successful consultant, speaker and writer.

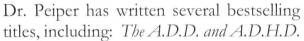

Throughout the years, his cutting-edge articles appeared in numerous medical journals and magazines. He also serves on the medical advisory board for several nutritional companies.

Dr. Peiper has written several bestselling titles, including: *The A.D.D. and A.D.H.D. Diet*, The *Secrets to Staying Young* and *New Hope for Serious Diseases*. He is a frequent guest speaker on radio and television programs. He even hosted his own shows, including the award-winning television show, "Partners in Healing."

NOTES:

NOTES:

Made in the USA
Monee, IL
17 April 2021

66080486R00031